Fire Cupping

A Beginner's 5-Step Quick Start Guide and Overview of Its Use Cases for Healing

mf

copyright © 2023 Felicity Paulman

All rights reserved No part of this book may be reproduced, or stored in a retrieval system, or transmitted in any form or by any means, electronic, mechanical, photocopying, recording, or otherwise, without express written permission of the publisher.

Disclaimer

By reading this disclaimer, you are accepting the terms of the disclaimer in full. If you disagree with this disclaimer, please do not read the guide.

All of the content within this guide is provided for informational and educational purposes only, and should not be accepted as independent medical or other professional advice. The author is not a doctor, physician, nurse, mental health provider, or registered nutritionist/dietician. Therefore, using and reading this guide does not establish any form of a physician-patient relationship.

Always consult with a physician or another qualified health provider with any issues or questions you might have regarding any sort of medical condition. Do not ever disregard any qualified professional medical advice or delay seeking that advice because of anything you have read in this guide. The information in this guide is not intended to be any sort of medical advice and should not be used in lieu of any medical advice by a licensed and qualified medical professional.

The information in this guide has been compiled from a variety of known sources. However, the author cannot attest to or guarantee the accuracy of each source and thus should not be held liable for any errors or omissions.

You acknowledge that the publisher of this guide will not be held liable for any loss or damage of any kind incurred as a result of this guide or the reliance on any information provided within this guide. You acknowledge and agree that you assume all risk and responsibility for any action you undertake in response to the information in this guide.

Using this guide does not guarantee any particular result (e.g., weight loss or a cure). By reading this guide, you acknowledge that there are no guarantees to any specific outcome or results you can expect.

All product names, diet plans, or names used in this guide are for identification purposes only and are the property of their respective owners. The use of these names does not imply endorsement. All other trademarks cited herein are the property of their respective owners.

Where applicable, this guide is not intended to be a substitute for the original work of this diet plan and is, at most, a supplement to the original work for this diet plan and never a direct substitute. This guide is a personal expression of the facts of that diet plan.

Where applicable, persons shown in the cover images are stock photography models and the publisher has obtained the rights to use the images through license agreements with third-party stock image companies.

Table of Contents

Introduction 7
What Is Fire Cupping? 10
    The Process 11
    The Benefits of Fire Cupping 12
    Use Cases 14
    Advantages of Fire Cupping 18
    Disadvantages of Fire Cupping 19
    Who should avoid fire cupping? 21
Different Techniques Used in Fire Cupping 23
    Dry Cupping 23
    Wet Cupping 23
    Massage Cupping 24
    Flash Cupping 25
    Needle Cupping 25
5 Step-Guide on Getting Started the Fire Cupping ... 27
    Step 1: Choose a Trained Professional 27
    Step 2: Select the Appropriate Technique: 28
    Step 3: Prepare Your Skin 29
    Step 4: Enjoy and Relax 29
    Step 5: Follow-Up Care 30
What Should You Expect During Fire Cupping Therapy Session 31
    Suction sensation 31
    Redness and bruising 32
    Relaxation 32
    Heightened sensitivity 33
Post-Therapy Care 34
    Things to Do After the Fire Cupping Therapy 34
    Things to Avoid After Fire Cupping Therapy 38

Side Effects of Fire Cupping Therapy	42
Conclusion	**46**
FAQ	**48**
References and Helpful Links	**51**

Introduction

Have you ever pondered the factors that contribute to the exceptional health of some individuals? Are you sick and weary of conventional treatments that only provide you with short-term relief? If this is the case, then you may find that fire cupping is the answer you've been seeking. This age-old method has been utilized for the promotion of healing and general well-being for a considerable amount of time. Now is the time to educate yourself on this fascinating treatment and the ways in which it can be of help to you.

More than 2,000 years have passed since the earliest documentation of fire cupping, which was performed in ancient Chinese medicine. Cupping is a form of alternative medicine that includes creating a vacuum inside of cups that are then placed on the patient's skin. The cups are often constructed of glass or bamboo. Because of the vacuum, the skin is drawn upward, which can increase circulation, boost blood flow, and reduce muscle tension. It has also been demonstrated that fire cupping can aid in the treatment of respiratory ailments, digestive conditions, and even mental health conditions.

Fire cupping could be exactly what the doctor ordered for you if you're seeking a natural and integrative way to improve your health. Fire cupping, in contrast to more conventional therapies such as medicine or surgery, is non-invasive and produces very few negative side effects. Taking charge of your own health and well-being is another important benefit of doing so. You can feel enhanced physical and mental health, more relaxation, and an overall sense of balance and harmony with regular fire cupping sessions. Fire cupping is a form of alternative medicine.

Are you ready to give the practice of fire cupping a shot? There are a variety of approaches you can take to incorporate this treatment into your overall wellness routine. You have the option of purchasing your own set of cups and practicing fire cupping on your own at home, or you can go to a professional practitioner who specializes in the practice. It is crucial to contact your healthcare practitioner before beginning any new treatment to ensure that the treatment will be safe for you to use.

In this guide, we will talk about the following in full detail:

- What is Fire Cupping
- How Does Fire Cupping Work
- Use Cases
- Benefits and Some Disadvantages Of Fire Cupping
- Different Techniques Used In Fire Cupping
- 5-Step Guide to Get Started with Fire Cupping

- What Should You Expect During the Fire Cupping
- Side Effects of Fire Cupping
- Things To Do and To Avoid After the Fire Cupping

Keep reading to learn more about fire cupping and whether it's right for you.

What Is Fire Cupping?

Fire cupping is a form of alternative medicine that has a long history of use and has been practiced for many years with the goal of improving one's general health. The procedure comprises placing glass cups on the patient's skin and applying heat in order to create a vacuum effect. This causes the tissue underneath to be pulled upwards as a result. It is standard practice to keep the cups in place for a few minutes, which generates a vacuum-like effect that, when appropriately exploited, can assist relaxation, alleviate discomfort, and enhance circulation. Leaving the cups in place for a few minutes also generates a vacuum-like effect.

Although the practice of fire cupping may appear to be a recent fad, its origins can be traced all the way back to ancient China, where it was practiced as a kind of traditional medicine. It was believed that fire cupping could treat a variety of illnesses, from headaches to respiratory difficulties, by increasing the body's energy flow, also known as qi, through various pressure spots on the skin.

Although modern fire cupping has adapted to include a variety of contemporary materials and methods, the fundamental ideas behind the practice have not changed. Fire cupping is a natural and holistic approach that is gaining popularity as a method of treating chronic pain, lowering stress, and boosting overall wellness. Many people are turning to this method.

The Process

Fire cupping is a technique that includes placing cups on the skin and utilizing fire to produce a vacuum within the cups, which then lifts the skin up and away from the cups. The suction action can assist in enhancing blood flow and circulation, lowering inflammation, easing muscle tension, and facilitating relaxation.

There are a few different approaches to cupping, the most common of which are dry cupping, wet cupping, and fire cupping. Using heat to generate a vacuum inside the cups, fire cupping is one of the most popular types. The cups are normally fashioned from glass or bamboo, and they are available in a variety of sizes to cater to specific regions of the body.

Before beginning the fire cupping treatment, the practitioner will first wash the region of the patient's skin that will be contacted by the cups. After that, an ignitable substance like alcohol is applied to the interior of the cup, and the flame is created by doing so.

The flame is promptly put out by laying the cup upside down on the skin, which puts out the flame. Because the air inside the cup is being forced to cool down and compress, this results in a negative pressure that pulls the skin upward and into the cup.

The Benefits of Fire Cupping

Fire cupping has been used to treat a range of physical and mental health conditions. Benefits include:

Increases blood flow and circulation

The process of fire cupping produces a vacuum within the cups, which draws the blood that has become stagnant to the surface. This results in improved blood circulation and the oxygenation of the tissues. An increase in blood flow can aid in the healing process, decrease inflammation, and provide pain relief.

Stimulates the immune system

Fire cupping can boost the immune system by enhancing the flow of lymphatic fluids, which in turn can have a stimulating effect on the immune system. This can assist the body in warding off infections, reducing inflammation, and boosting the immune system as a whole.

Promotes relaxation

Fire cupping is a calming technique that can help relieve tension and promote relaxation. It also helps with the promotion of relaxation. As a result of the therapy's ability to stimulate the parasympathetic nervous system, patients may experience less stress, enhanced sleep, and an overall increased sensation of calm.

Detoxifies the body

Fire cupping stimulates the lymphatic system, which in turn helps the body detoxify itself by removing waste products and impurities. The therapy has the potential to improve lymphatic drainage, which in turn can lead to enhanced liver function, enhanced digestion, and general cleansing.

Improves respiratory function

Fire cupping can help enhance lung function and treat respiratory conditions including asthma and bronchitis. The treatment has the potential to lessen inflammation in the lungs, assist in breaking up phlegm, and make breathing easier.

Enhances skin health

Fire cupping has been shown to improve skin quality, as well as lessen the appearance of cellulite and acne, by stimulating collagen synthesis and boosting blood flow to the skin. This results in an overall improvement in the health of the skin. In addition to these benefits, the therapy may also help reduce inflammation and improve the skin's overall health.

Use Cases

Here are some of the most common uses for fire cupping:

Pain relief

There is some evidence that suggests that fire cupping may be particularly beneficial in reducing the pain that is caused by muscle tension, soreness, and injury. The treatment is effective because it increases the flow of blood and circulation to the affected area. This, in turn, can help reduce inflammation and expedite the healing process.

Headaches and migraines

Increased blood flow to the head and neck area is one of the ways in which fire cupping can help alleviate headaches and migraines. In addition, the therapy may help reduce tension and increase relaxation, both of which are potential contributors to the aforementioned types of pain.

Fibromyalgia

People who suffer from fibromyalgia may find that fire cupping is beneficial for their illness because it can help ease the muscle pain and stiffness that are associated with this ailment. In addition, the therapy can help improve sleep quality and relaxation, both of which are essential for the management of fibromyalgia symptoms.

Sports injuries

Fire cupping is a treatment that can be beneficial for athletes who are struggling with sports injuries since it can help speed up the healing process while also reducing pain and inflammation. Athletes will be able to recover from their injuries more quickly and get back to their sport if the therapy improves their range of motion as well as their flexibility.

Digestive issues

People who suffer from digestive diseases like irritable bowel syndrome (IBS), constipation, or acid reflux may benefit from fire cupping. The therapy might help stimulate the digestive tract and enhance gut health, which might result in improved digestion and fewer symptoms.

Respiratory problems

People who suffer from respiratory conditions including asthma, bronchitis, and allergies may find relief from their symptoms through the practice of fire cupping. The treatment has the potential to enhance lung function and lower inflammation across the respiratory system, resulting in improved breathing and less discomfort.

Anxiety and stress

Fire cupping is a therapy that may be relaxing and peaceful, and it can help reduce the levels of both anxiety and tension in the body. The treatment activates the parasympathetic nervous system, which in turn leads to increased levels of relaxation and a lessening of sensations of tension or anxiety.

Skin conditions

Acne, eczema, and psoriasis are just some of the skin diseases that can be helped by fire cupping. This therapy works by improving blood flow and stimulating the elimination of toxins from the body, which in turn helps improve the quality of the skin. Additionally, the therapy can increase collagen formation, which results in skin that is both healthier and smoother.

High blood pressure

By enhancing circulation and blood flow, fire cupping can help lower high blood pressure. The therapy has the potential to help induce relaxation and lower levels of tension in the body, both of which can be factors that contribute to high blood pressure.

Chronic fatigue syndrome

Fire cupping may be beneficial for persons who suffer from chronic fatigue syndrome since it has the potential to promote blood flow and oxygenation of tissues, which in turn can lead to increased levels of energy. In addition, the therapy can help lower tension and improve relaxation, both of which are essential for the management of chronic fatigue syndrome symptoms.

Back pain

Fire cupping can assist enhance blood flow and circulation to the affected area, which can be a helpful therapy for reducing back pain. In addition to relieving stress in the muscles, the therapy can help reduce inflammation, which in turn results in less discomfort and increased mobility.

Menstrual cramps

Because fire cupping can assist increase blood flow and reduce inflammation in the pelvic area, it may be beneficial for women who are experiencing menstrual cramps. It is also possible for the therapy to induce relaxation and relieve tension in the body, which can result in a reduction in the discomfort experienced during menstruation.

Insomnia

Fire cupping is a calming technique that can help enhance the quality of sleep and relieve insomnia. The stimulation of the parasympathetic nervous system that can result from the therapy can lead to decreased levels of tension and improved sleep quality.

Advantages of Fire Cupping

Non-invasive

Fire cupping is a non-invasive treatment that does not involve the use of needles or incisions. After being positioned on the surface of the skin, the cups generate a vacuum that lifts and tightens the skin. Because of this, it is a more secure and less uncomfortable option than various other therapies.

Low-risk

Fire cupping is generally believed to be risk-free for most people and is associated with very few adverse effects. To reduce the likelihood of adverse outcomes, it is critical, however, to collaborate with an experienced professional and adhere to all applicable safety requirements.

Cost-effective

In comparison to many other holistic treatments, such as acupuncture or massage, fire cupping is a relatively inexpensive kind of treatment. Because it can be carried out in a short amount of time and requires only a small quantity of equipment, more individuals are able to participate in it.

Versatile

Fire cupping is an effective treatment for a wide range of illnesses, including pain and inflammation, as well as concerns with respiratory function and immune function. Its versatility lies in this fact. Additionally, it can be utilized as an alternative therapy in conjunction with traditional treatments.

Holistic approach

Fire cupping is an example of an alternative treatment that takes a holistic approach to health and wellness by focusing on the treatment of the full person rather than just the symptoms. Fire cupping can contribute to an improvement in general well-being since it brings about internal balance and harmony throughout the body.

Disadvantages of Fire Cupping

While fire cupping has many benefits, there are also some potential disadvantages to consider.

Skin irritation

Skin irritation is a potential side effect of fire cupping, especially for individuals who already have sensitive skin. Bruising may also result from the procedure. Some individuals may experience discomfort or even agony as a result of the suction effect that is produced by the cups.

Burns

Because fire cupping involves the use of heat, there is a possibility of suffering burns if the procedure is not carried out properly. Burns or blisters can result if the cups are kept on the skin for an extended period of time, as is sometimes the case.

Infection

There is a danger of infection if the cups are not adequately sanitized between uses or if they are put on injured skin. Additionally, there is a risk of infection if the cups are not thoroughly sterilized between usage. People who suffer from certain medical disorders or have immune systems that are already impaired may be more prone to infection.

Adverse effects

Dizziness, nausea, and fainting are only some of the adverse effects that have been reported in very isolated cases among persons who have undergone fire cupping therapy. These effects are often modest in nature and do not last for very long.

Insufficient evidence from scientific studies

Although there is some anecdotal evidence to support the use of fire cupping, there is insufficient data from scientific studies to back up either its usefulness or its safety.

Even though there is a risk involved with fire cupping, many people continue to find that it has significant positive effects on their bodies. Individuals can experience the advantages of fire cupping while limiting the hazards associated with the practices if they collaborate with a trained practitioner and adhere to proper safety standards.

Who should avoid fire cupping?

While fire cupping is generally safe, there are certain groups of individuals who should avoid the procedure or at least take extra caution when considering it. These include:

Pregnant women

Fire cupping is not recommended for pregnant women, especially in the first trimester. The therapy may stimulate contractions and increase the risk of miscarriage or premature labor.

People with skin conditions

Individuals with skin conditions like eczema, psoriasis, or open wounds should avoid fire cupping as it can worsen the condition or cause infection.

Those with bleeding disorders

People with bleeding disorders like hemophilia or thrombocytopenia should avoid fire cupping as it can increase the risk of bleeding or bruising.

Cancer patients

People undergoing cancer treatment or with a history of cancer should avoid fire cupping as it can interfere with chemotherapy or radiation therapy.

Anyone with a weakened immune system

Individuals with a weakened immune system due to illnesses like HIV/AIDS, or those taking immunosuppressive medications should avoid fire cupping as it can increase the risk of infection and other complications. It is important to consult with a healthcare provider before undergoing any complementary therapies.

So before starting fire cupping, it is recommended to consult a healthcare provider to determine if the therapy is safe and beneficial for you.

Different Techniques Used in Fire Cupping

There are several different techniques used in fire cupping, and each one can produce unique results. Here are some of the most popular methods:

Dry Cupping

Dry cupping, also known as fire cupping, is a technique that includes swiftly placing a cup on the skin after lighting a combustible substance, like alcohol or paper, that is contained within a cup. This is done in order to induce a cupping effect. As the fire dies out, the surrounding air begins to cool, which produces a vacuum that draws the skin closer to the surface of the body. It is thought that this will increase blood flow and help the healing process.

Wet Cupping

Because it can reach deeper layers of tissue than dry cupping can, wet cupping is a method that is gaining a lot of popularity these days. In this method, very fine cuts are first formed on the surface of the skin, and then cups are applied directly on top of these wounds. When the cup is heated, a vacuum is created inside of it, which draws blood from the cuts and collects it in the cup.

It is claimed that the suction created might assist the release of tight muscles and relieve discomfort in the body. Additionally, the blood that is collected in the cup might be utilized for diagnostic purposes after it has been analyzed. Although it is deemed safe when performed by a trained professional, wet cupping is not something that should be tried without first receiving the appropriate training.

Massage Cupping

Massage cupping combines aspects of traditional Chinese medicinal massage with the practice of fire cupping. In order to establish suction on the skin, requires the utilization of cups made of glass or plastic in conjunction with a hand-held pump.

This suction can lessen overall inflammation and the pain felt by muscles, in addition to increasing circulation and stimulating soft tissue. The treatment of pain and tension in the lower back, neck, and shoulders can benefit tremendously from the application of massage cupping. Patients suffering from persistent pain or tension may find great alleviation through the utilization of this approach, which is growing in popularity.

Flash Cupping

Flash cupping includes rapidly applying and removing the cup in order to provide a massaging-like effect on the patient. It is claimed that this approach will enhance circulation, lower inflammation, and relax muscles that are tight. It is also possible to utilize it to target specific pressure points, such as those surrounding joints, which, when done correctly, can help reduce stress and pain.

The practice of flash cupping, which is utilized frequently in traditional Chinese medicine, is widely recognized as safe. Before attempting to apply this method on your own, it is essential to seek the advice of a qualified expert, as it could result in bodily harm.

Needle Cupping

The method known as "needle cupping" is one in which acupuncture needles are inserted into a cup, and then a vacuum is created using the cup. It has been demonstrated that practicing this method can cause a release of endorphins, enhance blood circulation, lessen inflammation, and relax muscles that are tight.

It is frequently used to target the deeper layers of tissue, and it can be an effective treatment for chronic pain and stress if it is applied correctly. Needle cupping is a method of fire cupping that is both safe and effective; nevertheless, it should only be administered by an experienced practitioner.

Each of these approaches can be tailored to address a unique set of issues and can be applied to a variety of locations on the body; additionally, they are frequently combined with more conventional means of treatment. It is essential to keep in mind that fire cupping should never be done under the supervision of a qualified medical professional and always in an environment that is clean and risk-free.

5 Step-Guide on Getting Started the Fire Cupping

Fire cupping is a powerful healing technique that has been used for centuries in traditional medicine. It can help stimulate blood flow, reduce muscle tension, and promote overall health and wellness. If you are interested in trying fire cupping as a form of therapy, it is important to follow the steps below to ensure safety and maximize the benefits of the treatment.

Step 1: Choose a Trained Professional

If you decide to give fire cupping a try, it is absolutely necessary to find a skilled specialist who has considerable experience and has gone through intensive training. It is essential to get confirmation that the individual in question is familiar with the method in question and that they adhere to the appropriate safety standards.

You should look for a practitioner who is certified in traditional Chinese medicine or acupuncture, as this implies that they have had specialized training in the technique of fire cupping. In addition, it is important to check that the practitioner is qualified and knowledgeable by requesting references or testimonials from prior patients. This will contribute to ensuring the best possible results and the highest possible level of safety.

Step 2: Select the Appropriate Technique:

The next step is to select a method that is appropriate for the specific area of the body that is going to be treated as well as the outcome that is wanted. This decision should be made as soon as possible. The difference between the massage technique and the wet technique is that the massage technique involves moving the cups in a circular motion, whilst the wet technique involves placing a cotton ball that has been drenched in water over the area where the cups would be placed. The massage technique also involves rotating the cups around in a circular motion.

Needle cupping requires the use of acupuncture needles in addition to the cups, whereas flash cupping just entails the placement and removal of the cups very quickly for a brief amount of time. It is of the utmost importance to confer with a practitioner who has a significant amount of experience and can lead the selection of a treatment approach that is both safe and effective. This guarantees that the patient receives the highest possible level of comfort and benefit.

Step 3: Prepare Your Skin

The preparation of the skin in an appropriate manner constitutes the third step in the process. In this stage, you will first exfoliate the area with a mild cleanser, and then you will apply heated almond or coconut oil to create a seal between the cup and the body. This will ensure that the cup stays in place throughout the process.

In order to reduce the risk of getting scratched or burned, it is essential to keep fingernails cut and remove any jewelry that might be in the vicinity. This phase is essential in order to provide the patient with a therapy that is both safe and comfortable. If the practitioner takes the time to properly prepare the skin, they will be able to help encourage better suction and circulation, which will ultimately lead to more effective results.

Step 4: Enjoy and Relax

As soon as the skin has been adequately prepped, it is time to position the cups. Before beginning the suctioning process, the practitioner will heat the cup with either a lighter or a cotton ball that has been drenched in alcohol. When installing each cup, the practitioner needs to go slowly and carefully in order to maximize the patient's level of comfort and minimize the risk of injury.

In addition, during this procedure, they should pay close attention to any input provided by the patient so that they can make appropriate adjustments. In order to maximize the efficacy of the treatment while also reducing any potential hazards, this phase calls for patience and attention.

Step 5: Follow-Up Care

After the treatment with fire cupping, it is essential to receive aftercare in order to obtain the greatest possible benefit and level of comfort. This may entail taking a warm bath or shower, as well as drinking plenty of water, in order to assist in relaxing the muscles.

Stretching gently can also help reduce any stress or stiffness that you may be experiencing. In addition, compresses made of herbs like chamomile or lavender can be used to the marks left by the cupping to assist reduce any swelling or bruising that may have occurred.

If you follow these instructions, you will be able to ensure that your treatment with fire cupping is both safe and effective. Fire cupping is a technique that has been shown to effectively promote overall health and wellness by increasing blood flow, reducing muscle tension, and promoting overall health and wellness.

When engaging in this therapy, it is essential to keep in mind that it is imperative to always seek the guidance of a skilled practitioner. You may get all of the benefits that fire cupping has to offer with the right level of care and technique.

What Should You Expect During Fire Cupping Therapy Session

Fire cupping therapy is an ancient practice that involves placing cups on the skin and creating a vacuum to promote healing. Here's what you can expect during a typical fire cupping therapy session:

Suction sensation

It is usual for the patient to experience a strong suction sensation once the cups have been placed on the patient's skin during a session of fire cupping. This sensation may last for several minutes. This is one of the many advantages that come with undergoing the procedure. Perhaps while the vacuum that is created inside the cups could cause a little bit of discomfort or perhaps a small bit of suffering, it should not be intolerable.

A deeper level of relaxation and a reduction in stress levels can be achieved with the use of suction, which helps to loosen tight muscles and fascia. Additionally, it assists in the relaxation of tense muscles. It is imperative that you communicate with the practitioner as soon as the sensation of suction becomes intolerable at any point during the treatment. This will allow the practitioner to either adjust the amount of pressure that is being applied or move the cups to a different position on the body.

Redness and bruising

During a session of fire cupping, it is anticipated that the patient would experience an increase in the flow of blood to the areas that are being cupped with fire. Patients who go through with this treatment run the risk of experiencing bruising and/or redness in the areas of their bodies where the cups were applied while the process was being carried out.

On the other hand, considering that this is a normal reaction, there is no need to be concerned about it in any way. This demonstrates that the treatment was successful in improving the patient's circulation and creating general improvements to their health. Within a few days, the patient will typically see a reduction in the redness and bruising, at which point they will feel revitalized and rejuvenated. This will be the case in most cases.

Relaxation

A session of fire cupping, which has been compared to the sensation of having a massage, is known to bring about a profound sense of relaxation in the person who receives the treatment. When the heated cups are put in specific areas of the body, they produce a vacuum that raises the skin as well as the underlying muscle tissue. This results in a more youthful appearance.

This technique is helpful for relieving stress in the muscles as well as increasing blood flow and circulation in the lymphatic system. Additionally, there is a possibility that the process will increase the synthesis of endorphins, which are neurotransmitters that can lift one's mood and contribute to an overall sense of well-being. In addition, the warmth of the cups can induce a sense of comfort, which is further enhanced by the light suction that is administered during the treatment.

Heightened sensitivity

Individuals may experience increased sensitivity in the areas that are being treated with fire cupping, which may lead to a heightened awareness of the feelings that are occurring within the body. Fire cupping is a traditional Chinese medicine technique. This takes place as a consequence of the increased blood flow to particular areas, which might stimulate nerve activity and assist the body in its ability to mend itself.

In general, fire cupping therapy can be an effective method that is also quite calming, with the added benefit of promoting healing and improving overall health. Before attempting any new treatments, it is crucial to discuss any concerns with a qualified medical expert.

Post-Therapy Care

Once the fire cupping therapy is completed, it is important to take care of your body to ensure that its effects are maximized and that you don't suffer from any negative side effects.

Things to Do After the Fire Cupping Therapy

It is essential to follow the recommended aftercare procedures following a session of fire cupping in order to guarantee that the body reaps the full advantages of this age-old form of alternative medicine. If individuals follow these guidelines, they will be able to maximize the benefits and reduce the risk of any potential adverse effects.

Drink plenty of water

It is essential to drink enough water after your Fire Cupping Therapy session in order to reap the full advantages of the treatment. It is highly recommended that you drink a lot of water because it assists the body in flushing out dangerous toxins and restores the fluids that were lost while the process is taking place.

This practice is helpful for cleansing the body of toxins, reducing dehydration, and enhancing general wellness. In order to speed up the recovery process, it is recommended that one drink at least 8 to 10 glasses of water each day.

Rest and relax

It is imperative that you get enough rest and give your body time to heal after undergoing fire cupping therapy. This means refraining from activities that are physically taxing and getting sufficient amounts of rest. When this is done, the body is given enough time to mend naturally, which lessens the likelihood of experiencing any discomfort or tiredness as a result of the therapy.

In order to assist the body in refueling itself, it is also advisable to consume a substantial amount of water and a meal that is rich in nutrients. A warm bath will also help to relax the muscles and reduce any soreness that you may be experiencing. A proper amount of relaxation and care given after treatment with fire cupping will help enhance the advantages of the treatment and ensure a speedy recovery.

Eat healthy foods

Following treatment with fire cupping, you should eat meals that are rich in nutrients and give a good amount of antioxidants, vitamins, and minerals. These should be consumed as soon as possible. This will help the body heal at a faster rate while it recovers from the injury.

Consuming fresh fruits and vegetables, proteins that are low in fat, cereals that are whole, and meals that are high in healthy fats are some of the things that are recommended to do so. These foods can provide the body with the nutrients and energy it requires for the process of healing, which is something the body demands.

Apply heat or ice

After undergoing the Fire Cupping Therapy treatment, you should apply either heat or ice to the area that was cupped in order to alleviate any discomfort that may have been brought on by the procedure. It is imperative that you seek the guidance of an experienced medical professional in order to determine which method will be the most successful in alleviating pain or inflammation.

While heat causes an increase in blood flow, cold brings down swelling. Both approaches have the potential to alleviate pain and speed up the healing process. When administering heat or ice, it is imperative to exercise caution and strictly adhere to the time intervals that are prescribed in order to avoid causing injury.

Take a warm bath

After undergoing Fire Cupping therapy, it is advisable to take a warm bath in order to ease any discomfort or soreness that may have been caused by the treatment. Because Epsom salts have been shown to reduce inflammation, adding some to your bathwater is a good idea to take advantage of its anti-inflammatory properties.

The body will have a soothing effect as a result of the warm temperature of the water, and any aches and pains in the muscles will be alleviated as a result of this. The therapeutic advantages of the therapy might be increased by taking time to rest and unwind before or after the session.

Wear loose clothing

Following treatment with fire cupping, it is recommended that the treated region be covered with clothes that are both loose and comfortable in order to avoid any irritation or pain. The restriction of blood flow caused by wearing clothing that is too tight might also slow down the healing process. It is essential that you continue to use this preventative step for a few days following the therapy in order to attain the best possible outcomes.

Monitor the cupping marks

After receiving treatment with fire cupping, you should closely monitor the circular bruises that emerge on their skin in order to guarantee that the wounds are healing correctly. If there are any signs that an infection may be present, such as an increase in discomfort or abnormal darkness, it is vital to get medical help as soon as possible. Delaying treatment could result in serious complications. It is essential to engage in healthy self-care practices after finishing treatment in order to lower the likelihood of experiencing any complications.

Things to Avoid After Fire Cupping Therapy

After fire cupping, there are certain things that individuals should avoid to promote healing and prevent any potential complications. Here are some things to avoid after fire cupping:

Strenuous exercise

It is recommended that you wait at least twenty-four hours after undergoing fire cupping therapy before indulging in severe physical activities. Exerting oneself beyond what is comfortable may slow down the healing process and lead to muscle strain or injury if the person continues to push themselves. When given the opportunity to relax, the body is able to recoup more completely and attain greater overall results.

Exposure to extreme temperatures

It is recommended that individuals avoid exposure to severe temperatures after undergoing fire cupping therapy in order to promote optimal healing. This means avoiding temperatures that rapidly shift, such as those found in hot saunas and cold swimming pools, as this can shock the body and potentially slow down the healing process. In order to get the outcomes you want from the treatment, it is absolutely necessary to make maintaining a peaceful and nurturing atmosphere a top priority.

Alcohol and caffeine

After completing fire-cupping therapy, you should abstain from consuming any alcohol or caffeine for at least 24 hours. Because of the dehydrating effect that these chemicals can have on the body, the treatment's benefits may not be maximized to their full potential. Because the body of the patient will require sustenance and rehydration after undergoing this treatment, it is imperative that they abstain from drinking alcoholic beverages and caffeine during this time.

Additionally, the consumption of alcoholic beverages and beverages containing caffeine might impede the natural healing process of the body, diminishing the efficacy of the treatment. Because of this, if you want to get the most out of your fire-cupping therapy session, it is strongly advised that you abstain from eating these substances.

Showers or baths immediately

Because the skin may be sensitive shortly after fire cupping, you should avoid taking hot showers or baths. An excessively high water temperature might be a source of discomfort and irritation. If you want the healing process to go as smoothly and quickly as possible, you should wait at least two to three hours before getting in the shower.

This amount of time must pass in order to provide the skin with sufficient opportunity to recuperate following the treatment. After the allotted amount of time has passed, it is strongly suggested that you take a bath in cool or tepid water to alleviate any additional discomfort.

Scratching or picking at the cupping marks

It is essential to fight the temptation to scratch or pick at the circular markings left behind by the fire cupping therapy in order to facilitate a speedy recovery after the treatment. These kinds of acts might irritate the skin and slow down the healing process, producing unneeded pain and discomfort in the affected area.

Therefore, it is better to let the marks heal on their own nature and avoid any further aggravation by wearing clothing that does not fit snugly and avoiding activities that may cause the affected regions to be rubbed against.

Sun exposure

Following a session of fire cupping, it is advised to stay out of the sun for as long as possible so as not to risk getting a sunburn or further irritating the skin. In the event that sun exposure cannot be avoided, it is critical to wear protective clothing and apply sunscreen to the region that will be cupped.

Massage or chiropractic adjustments

It is essential to refrain from getting any kind of massage or chiropractic adjustments to the afflicted regions for at least 24 hours after receiving Fire Cupping Therapy. This will ensure that you receive the full benefits of the treatment. These kinds of interventions might not only irritate the skin but also slow down the healing process, which can result in additional discomfort and a longer period of time spent recovering.

Applying oils or lotions

It is important to wait at least 24 hours following a fire cupping therapy session before putting any oils or lotions on the skin. This will help prevent any additional discomfort or irritation from occurring. In spite of the fact that it is a frequent practice, topical products might make the skin more sensitive after treatment, which can make the problem much worse. Instead, you should focus on letting your skin recover in its natural state by allowing it to breathe and heal.

Individuals may ensure that the healing process is not hindered and that they are able to get the full advantages of this ancient therapy by avoiding these things after having fire cupping performed on them.

Side Effects of Fire Cupping Therapy

Fire cupping is a safe and effective form of therapy when performed by a trained professional. However, some potential side effects can occur after the treatment.

The following side effects include:

Cupping marks

It is normal for patients who undergo fire cupping therapy to have the side effect of the appearance of cup markings. These marks can last anywhere from a few days to a week and can appear in a variety of colors. However, they are not painful and should not be considered harmful. They are a sign of an enhanced circulation of blood in the affected area, which is beneficial to the healing process.

Marks of cupping are a natural reaction to the vacuum effect induced by fire cupping, and their presence is an indication that the therapy was successful. Compresses made of herbal ingredients can reduce the appearance of any swelling or bruising caused by the markings. It is essential to have faith in the curative effects of fire cupping and to not be intimidated by the seemingly harmful markings that may be left behind.

Soreness or discomfort

An area that has been treated with fire cupping may feel sore or uncomfortable as a potential adverse consequence of the treatment. This is typically the result of improved circulation as well as the stimulation of the muscle tissue that takes place throughout the therapy.

Even though this soreness is completely natural and should go away after a few days, some people can experience it more strongly than others do. As a consequence of this, it is essential to convey any discomfort to the therapist, who may then suggest an herbal compress or other therapies in order to reduce the level of pain and swelling.

Nausea

The use of fire cupping therapy has been known to occasionally cause nausea as a side effect. This is because of the abrupt increase in circulation, which, along with the stimulation of muscles, can lead to an imbalance of chemicals in the body.

Additionally, it is recommended that you get medical assistance in the event that the symptoms continue or worsen. It is possible to reduce the risk of experiencing any adverse effects from fire cupping therapy by ensuring that the appropriate aftercare and technique are followed.

Fatigue

The fatigue that can result from fire cupping typically sets in a few hours after the treatment has been completed. This is because the muscles are being stimulated more, which leads to a fall in oxygen levels and an increase in the generation of lactic acid. The increased circulation is also to blame.

After receiving treatment, it is essential to get plenty of rest, drink a lot of water, and refrain from engaging in physically taxing activities for at least a few hours. In addition, getting the recommended amount of sleep each night and maintaining a balanced diet can assist in the reduction of weariness and the promotion of healing. To get the most out of your fire cupping therapy session, it is imperative that you practice proper aftercare.

Numbness or tingling

There is a possibility that the area that was treated with fire cupping will feel numb or tingly once the treatment is finished. This effect is the result of the cups creating a vacuum, which stimulates nerves and enhances circulation. The effect is achieved by the cups' suction. Because of this, it is possible that the individual will experience a sensation of numbness or tingling that may continue for several hours after the treatment has been carried out.

To reduce the amount of rubbing and irritation that takes place on the skin, it is vital to make use of high-quality oil such as jojoba or grapeseed. In addition, it is of the utmost importance to adhere to the proper procedures in order to assist in minimizing any potential discomfort that may be created by the treatment.

Emotional release

It is possible to experience a release of pent-up emotions as a side effect of cupping therapy, which includes placing heated cups on the skin to generate a suction effect. This may cause individuals to have intensified feelings, which is a healthy indicator that the treatment is having the desired effect. It is essential to keep in mind that the emotional release usually passes within a few hours and is a completely natural element of the body's process of healing.

It is claimed that fire cupping can increase the flow of energy throughout the body, which can result in emotional breakthroughs and a sense of well-being for the patient. Even while the emotional outpouring could be overpowering at first, many people find that it is a life-changing event that brings them closer to their feelings and improves their overall health.

It's important to remember that these side effects are typically mild and short-lived. However, if they persist or worsen, individuals should seek medical attention. It's also important to note that individuals may react differently to cupping therapy, and what works well for one person may not work as well for another. As with any natural healing practice, it's important to listen to the body and communicate openly with a healthcare professional.

Conclusion

Congratulations! You've reached the end of our Fire Cupping Guide. We really hope that you have been provided with all of the information necessary to complete this ancient Chinese ritual in a manner that is both secure and fruitful. Bear in mind that, despite the fact that, at first glance, fire cupping may appear to be an intimidating technique, it is actually a quite straightforward and gratifying method that can help ease pain and promote healing in a broad variety of ailments.

You now know that there are many distinct types of cupping techniques, such as dry cupping, wet cupping, and fire cupping, among others. It is essential to select the strategy that is most suited to meet your specific requirements, as each of these approaches comes with a distinct set of advantages and disadvantages. In addition, it is vital to take the appropriate safety precautions when practicing fire cupping, such as utilizing cups of high quality, performing the procedure in an area that is clean and hygienic, and keeping a steady hand.

We hope that at the end of this book, you have a better understanding of the wider range of benefits that this technique offers, in addition to the technical components of fire cupping that you have learned. When it comes to reducing stress and enhancing overall health, fire cupping can be a very effective strategy. This can help you feel more energized, focused, and balanced by inducing relaxation, lowering inflammation, and boosting circulation.

Therefore, get over your apprehension and give fire cupping a shot! Fire cupping is an ancient practice that has several potential health benefits, including the reduction of pain and inflammation, the stimulation of the immune system, and a sense of calm and relaxation at the end of a long day.

FAQ

What exactly is a fire cup?

The ancient Chinese technique of fire cupping is a form of alternative medicine that includes applying glass cups to the patient's skin and then using fire to create a vacuum there. This vacuum pushes the skin as well as the muscular tissue into the cup, which in turn helps to enhance blood flow and provides some relief from pain.

How does it work?

Fire cupping creates a vacuum that helps to enhance blood flow and circulation, which in turn can assist in alleviating pain. In addition to this, it helps to break up scar tissue and loosen up muscles that are tight.

What are the advantages of doing so?

Fire cupping has been shown to have numerous potential health benefits, including the reduction of pain, the increase of circulation, and the breaking up of scar tissue. In addition, it is believed that the removal of toxins from the body through the use of fire cupping can help enhance general health.

How long does it take?

The duration of a session of fire cupping is typically around 15 minutes. However, the number of cups that are utilized as well as the amount of time that each cup is left in place will change according to the requirements of the individual.

Is it painful?

Fire cupping is not normally painful, however, some people may feel a little burning sensation when the cups are first placed on the skin. However, the majority of people do not report any pain during the process. As the vacuum is generated, you should notice that this sensation disappears relatively soon.

Are there any potential adverse reactions?

The practice of fire cupping is not typically associated with any adverse effects. On the other hand, after a session, some people find that the area where the cups have been placed becomes bruised or uncomfortable. These adverse effects are often not severe and should go away within a few days' time at the latest.

How frequently should I carry it out?

Regarding the question of how frequently one should participate in fire cupping therapy, there is no clear answer.

However, in order for people to see the maximum outcomes, it is normally recommended that they have treatments two to three times per week.

References and Helpful Links

Sage Health. (2016, August 22). Fire Cupping: Insights and Benefits. Sage Health Wellness Center. https://sagehealthonline.com/fire-cupping-insights-and-benefits/

Criterion Wellness Clinic. (2022, October 19). Traditional Chinese Fire Cupping - Break Up Stagnation & Congestion. https://www.criterionwellness.ca/services/traditional-chinese-fire-cupping/

Shaw, J. (n.d.). Fire Cupping - Energize Health - Physiotherapy and Chiropractic Clinic in Calgary. Energize Health - Physiotherapy and Chiropractic Clinic in Calgary. https://energizehealth.ca/about/careers/south-opportunities/16-blog/31-fire-cupping.html

Weatherall, D. (2006). Science and Technology for Disease Control: Past, Present, and Future. Disease Control Priorities in Developing Countries - NCBI Bookshelf. https://www.ncbi.nlm.nih.gov/books/NBK11740/

Fire Cupping. (n.d.). RadCo Rehab. https://radcomassage.com/fire-cupping

Marcin, A. (2023, May 10). What Is Cupping Therapy? Healthline. https://www.healthline.com/health/cupping-therapy

www.ingramcontent.com/pod-product-compliance
Lightning Source LLC
LaVergne TN
LVHW051925060526
838201LV00062B/4688